LOW FAT HIGH FIBER

DIET PREP

COOKBOOK FOR BEGINNERS

Over 2000 Days of Healthy, Simple, and Delicious Recipes Ready under 30 minutes

JANE SCOTT rdn

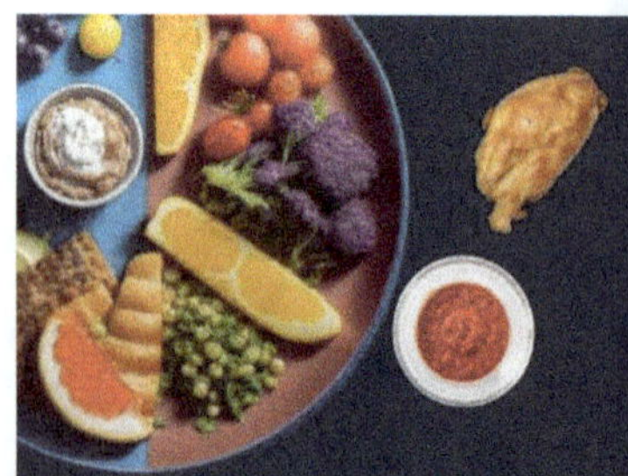

LOW FAT HIGH FIBER
DIET PREP
COOKBOOK
FOR BEGINNERS

Over 2000 Days of Healthy, Simple, and Delicious Recipes Ready under 30 minutes.

BONUS IMAGES INCLUDED

2000 DAYS
OF LOW FAT HIGH FIBER
FLAVORS

JANE SCOTT rdn

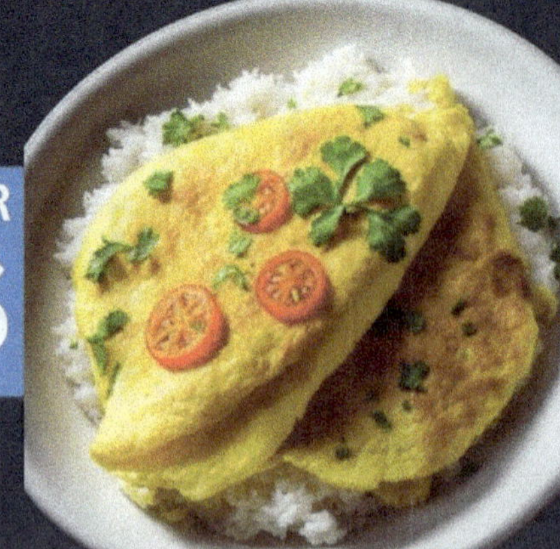

Table of Contents

Introduction to Low Fat High Fiber Diet Cookbook

In the constantly changing world of nutrition and dietary choices, the low-fat, high-fiber diet shines as a model of health-conscious eating, providing a balanced and sustainable path to wellness. This dietary approach focuses on two key principles: lowering fat intake and increasing fiber-rich food consumption. As more people look for nutritional strategies to enhance overall well-being, the low-fat, high-fiber diet distinguishes itself with its ability to address various health issues, ranging from weight management to heart health and more.

A Holistic Approach to Wellness

At its essence, the low-fat, high-fiber diet transcends being a mere temporary regimen and represents a lifestyle shift with lasting health benefits. This dietary approach focuses on reducing dietary fats, particularly saturated and trans fats, while simultaneously incorporating abundant fiber from plant-based sources. This balance aims to optimize nutrient intake and reduce the risks associated with excessive fat consumption.

The low-fat aspect of the diet is rooted in the recognition that not all fats are the same. While certain fats are necessary for bodily functions, an excess of saturated and trans fats can lead to health issues such as high cholesterol and cardiovascular diseases. Therefore, this diet encourages the consumption of healthier fats found in nuts, seeds, avocados, and fatty fish, while limiting processed and fried foods.

The high-fiber component of the diet offers numerous benefits. Fiber, an indigestible carbohydrate in plant foods, is crucial for digestive health, weight management, and preventing chronic diseases. Emphasizing high-fiber foods like fruits, vegetables, whole grains, legumes, and nuts provides a diverse range of nutrients and promotes a sense of fullness, aiding in weight control.

A significant advantage of the low-fat, high-fiber diet is its versatility and adaptability. It is not a rigid plan but a flexible framework that can accommodate various dietary preferences. Whether someone prefers a vegetarian or omnivorous diet, the principles can be tailored to fit personal tastes, making it an inclusive option for many individuals.

The benefits of adopting a low-fat, high-fiber diet extend beyond weight management. Numerous studies suggest that this dietary pattern may reduce the risk of chronic conditions such as cardiovascular diseases, type 2 diabetes, and certain cancers. Emphasizing whole, nutrient-dense foods aligns with broader heart-healthy lifestyle recommendations, and the inclusion of fiber-rich foods can positively affect cholesterol levels, blood sugar regulation, and digestive health.

Weight management is a central focus of the low-fat, high-fiber diet. The combination of reduced fat intake and increased fiber consumption creates a calorie-friendly environment, fostering a sense of fullness and satisfaction with fewer calories. This sustainable approach can help those aiming to achieve or maintain a healthy weight, avoiding short-term fads or restrictive measures.

Notably, the low-fat, high-fiber diet supports cardiovascular health. Reducing saturated and trans fats, along with the cholesterol-lowering effects of soluble fiber, contributes to a heart-protective dietary pattern. As cardiovascular diseases remain a leading cause of global morbidity and mortality, adopting heart-healthy eating habits becomes increasingly important.

Moreover, the low-fat, high-fiber diet aligns with contemporary nutritional guidelines that emphasize the importance of plant-based foods. As plant-forward diets gain recognition for their environmental sustainability and health benefits, the emphasis on fruits, vegetables, whole grains, and legumes in this dietary approach resonates with broader shifts towards a more plant-centric eating paradigm.

The potential impact of the low-fat, high-fiber diet extends to metabolic health, particularly in the context of insulin sensitivity and type 2 diabetes prevention. Fiber-rich foods contribute to steady blood sugar levels, and the overall nutritional profile of the diet may play a role in reducing the risk of developing insulin resistance—a precursor to type 2 diabetes.

In conclusion, the low-fat, high-fiber diet emerges as a compelling and adaptable approach to nutrition, offering a roadmap to improved health and well-being. Its principles, rooted in evidence-based nutrition, provide a foundation for sustainable dietary habits that address not only weight management but also broader health concerns. By reducing the intake of unhealthy fats and embracing the wealth of nutrients found in high-fiber foods, individuals can embark on a journey towards a balanced and nourishing lifestyle— one that promotes longevity, supports cardiovascular health, and contributes to the overall vitality of body and mind.

Foods to Eat and Foods to Avoid on Low Fat High Fiber Diet

Striking the balance between minimizing fat and maximizing fiber can feel like walking a tightrope. But worry not, intrepid explorer! This book equips you with the knowledge and resources to navigate the delicious world of a low-fat, high-fiber diet. Buckle up as we unveil the foods to embrace and those to politely decline, all while keeping your taste buds happy and your gut singing.

Foods to Eat

Plant Powerhouse: Fruits and vegetables reign supreme here. Leafy greens like kale, spinach, and arugula pack a fiber punch while being virtually fat-free. Don't shy away from colorful veggies like broccoli, bell peppers, and carrots; they're vitamin and fiber goldmines. And fruits like berries, apples, and pears offer sweetness and fiber without the fat overload.

- **Whole Grain Warriors:** Swap refined grains for their whole-grain counterparts. Brown rice, quinoa, whole-wheat bread, and oatmeal are champions of both fiber and complex carbohydrates, keeping you feeling full and energized. Bonus points for getting creative with ancient grains like amaranth and teff!

- **Legume Legends:** Beans, lentils, and chickpeas are your fiber and protein besties. Toss them into salads, soups, and curries, or whip up a hummus feast. Just remember to soak and cook them well to avoid digestive discomfort.

- **Nutty Delights:** Nuts and seeds, like almonds, walnuts, and chia seeds, are tiny nutrition powerhouses. Sprinkle them on salads, yogurt, or homemade granola for a fiber and healthy fat boost. Moderation is key, though, as they can be calorie-dense.

- **Hydration Heroes:** Don't underestimate the power of water! Staying hydrated promotes digestion and helps your body utilize fiber effectively. Aim for eight glasses of water daily and enjoy herbal teas or low-sugar fruit-infused water for variety.

Foods to Gently Sidestep

- Fat Kings: Fatty meats like marbled steaks, sausages, and processed meats are high in saturated fat and cholesterol, which you want to limit. Lean protein sources like skinless chicken breasts, fish, and tofu are your low-fat allies.

- **Dairy Dilemmas:** Opt for low-fat or fat-free dairy products like milk, yogurt, and cheese. Full-fat versions, while delicious, can quickly bump up your daily fat intake.

- **Fried Fantasies:** Fried foods, whether sweet or savory, are laden with unhealthy fats and low in fiber. Choose baked, grilled, or steamed cooking methods instead to keep your heart and gut happy.

- **Sugar Sirens:** Sugar-laden treats like cookies, cakes, and candies offer empty calories and minimal fiber. Satisfy your sweet tooth with naturally sweet fruits or unsweetened dark chocolate in moderation.

- **Hidden Fat Traps:** Watch out for sneaky sources of fat like creamy salad dressings, pre-made sauces, and processed snacks. Read food labels carefully and choose low-fat alternatives whenever possible.

Creating a Delicious Low-Fat, High-Fiber Feast

Now that you know your food friends and foes, let's assemble a delectable plate! Start with a base of leafy greens or whole-grain carbohydrates. Add a rainbow of vegetables, protein like grilled chicken or lentils, and sprinkle with chopped nuts or seeds for a satisfying crunch. Don't forget a drizzle of heart-healthy olive oil or a squeeze of lemon for extra flavor.

Beyond the Plate:

Remember, healthy eating is a lifestyle, not just a diet. Stay active with regular exercise, manage stress, and prioritize sleep. These holistic approaches will further optimize your well-being and support your low-fat, high-fiber journey.

Tools for Your Journey:

Meal planning apps: Plan your meals for the week with apps like Mealime or Yummly.

Grocery delivery services: Save time and energy with grocery delivery services.

Recipe websites: Discover endless recipe inspiration for low-fat, high-fiber meals on websites like Cookie and Kate or Minimalist Baker.

The Bottom Line

Embracing a low-fat, high-fiber diet doesn't have to be bland or restrictive. With the right knowledge and delicious recipe hacks, you can nourish your body, satisfy your taste buds, and pave the way for a healthier, happier you. So, raise a glass of water to your newfound foodie skills and embark on this flavor-packed adventure!

Remember, this is just a starting point. Always consult with a healthcare professional or registered dietitian for personalized dietary advice specific to your needs and health conditions.

Low Fat High Fiber Diet Cookbook

Side Dishes

Roasted Vegetable Medley

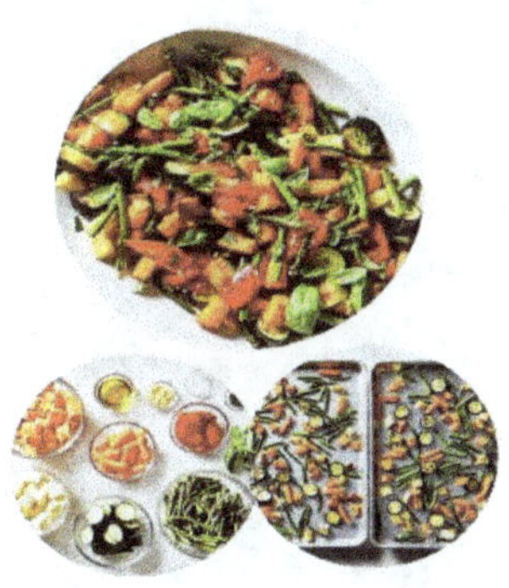

Ingredients

2 tablespoons olive oil, divided

1 large yam, peeled and cut into 1 inch pieces

1 large parsnip, peeled and cut into 1 inch pieces

1 cup baby carrots

1 zucchini, cut into 1 inch slices

1 bunch fresh asparagus, trimmed and cut into 1 inch pieces

½ cup roasted red peppers, cut into 1-inch pieces

¼ cup chopped fresh basil

2 cloves garlic, minced

½ teaspoon kosher salt

½ teaspoon ground black pepper

Directions

Gather all ingredients. Preheat the oven to 425 degrees F (220 degrees C). Grease two baking sheets with 1/2 tablespoon olive oil each.

Place yam, parsnip, and carrots onto the baking sheets.

Bake in the preheated oven for 30 minutes, then add zucchini and asparagus, and drizzle with remaining 1 tablespoon olive oil. Continue baking until all the vegetables are tender, about 30 minutes more.

Once tender, remove from the oven, and allow to cool for 30 minutes on the baking sheet.

Toss roasted peppers together with basil, garlic, salt, and pepper in a large bowl until combined.

Add the roasted vegetables, and toss to mix. Serve at room temperature or cold.

Quinoa and Chickpea Salad

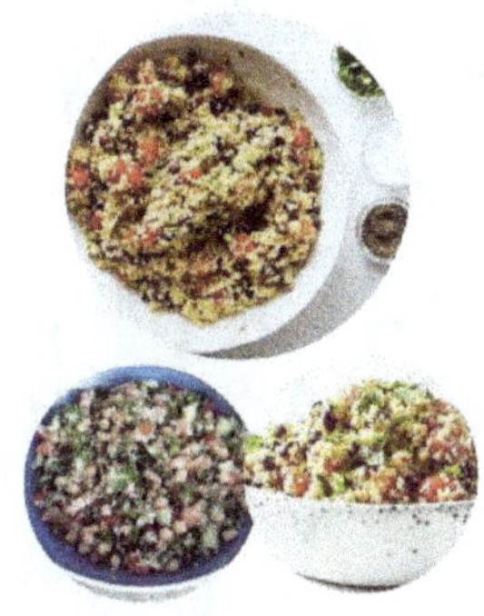

Ingredients

1 cup water

½ cup quinoa

1 cup rinsed canned chickpeas

1 cup diced tomatoes

1 cup diced cucumber

1 cup chopped green onions

1 cup chopped fresh parsley

3 tablespoons lemon juice

2 tablespoons extra-virgin olive oil

3 cloves garlic, minced

2 teaspoons chopped fresh mint

½ teaspoon salt

½ teaspoon ground black pepper

Directions

Bring water and quinoa to a boil in a saucepan. Reduce heat to medium-low, cover, and simmer until quinoa is tender, 15 to 20 minutes. Set aside to cool.

Combine chickpeas, tomatoes, cucumber, green onions, and parsley in a large bowl. Stir in cooled quinoa.

Mix lemon juice, olive oil, garlic, mint, salt, and pepper together in a separate small bowl. Pour over quinoa mixture; toss to combine.

Spicy Baked Sweet Potato Fries

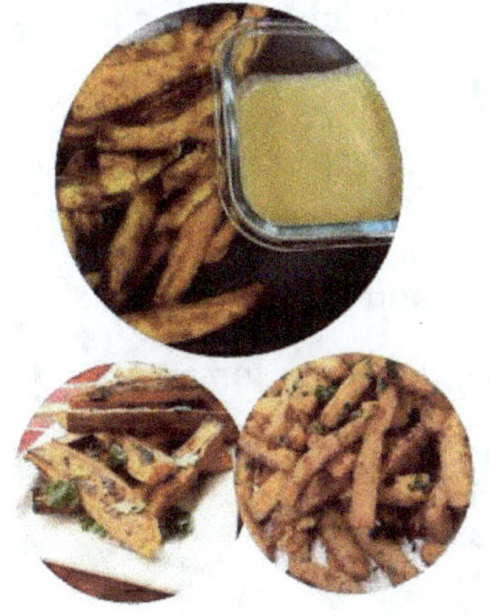

Ingredients

6 sweet potatoes, cut into French fries

2 tablespoons canola oil

3 tablespoons taco seasoning mix

¼ teaspoon cayenne pepper

Directions

Preheat the oven to 425 degrees F (220 degrees C).

In a plastic bag, combine the sweet potatoes, canola oil, taco seasoning, and cayenne pepper. Close and shake the bag until the fries are evenly coated. Spread the fries out in a single layer on two large baking sheets.

Bake for 30 minutes, or until crispy and brown on one side. Turn the fries over using a spatula, and cook for another 30 minutes, or until they are all crispy on the outside and tender inside. Thinner fries may not take as lon

Lentils and Rice with TVP

This lentil and rice with TVP (textured vegetable protein) recipe is cooked in broth with onion and spices.

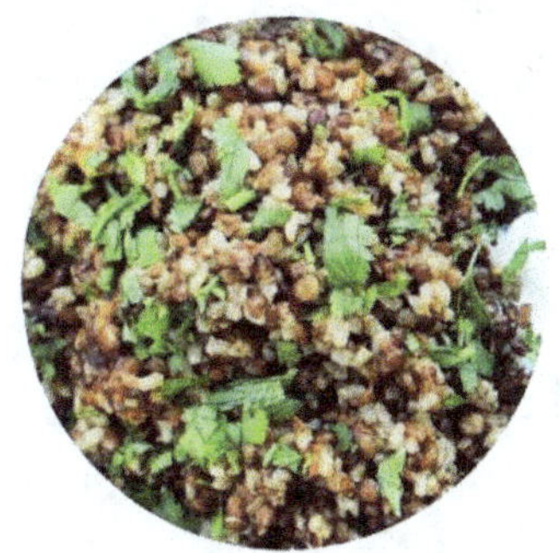

Ingredients

5 ½ cups water, divided

1 cup brown lentils

1 ½ teaspoons olive oil

1 medium onion, chopped

1 cup long grain white rice

½ cup texturized vegetable protein (TVP)

2 tablespoons dried parsley flakes

4 ½ teaspoons chicken bouillon granules

1 teaspoon curry powder

1 teaspoon ground cumin

ground black pepper to taste

Directions

Combine 3 cups water and lentils in a large saucepan; bring to a boil. Reduce heat to medium-low and simmer uncovered for 10 minutes.

Meanwhile, heat olive oil in a skillet over medium heat. Cook and stir onion in hot oil until translucent, about 5 minutes. Set aside.

Once lentils have simmered for 10 minutes, stir in remaining 2 1/2 cups water, cooked onion, rice, TVP, parsley, bouillon, curry powder, and cumin. Return to a boil over high heat, then remove from heat, cover, and let stand undisturbed for 20 minutes.

Season with pepper and stir before serving.

Roasted Brussels Sprouts with Garlic

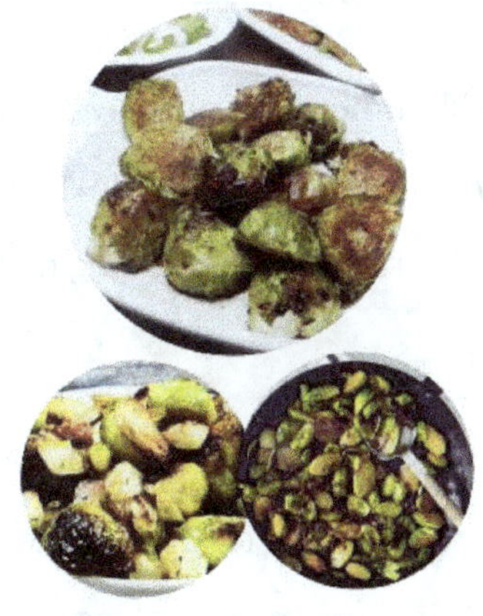

Ingredients

6 tablespoons olive oil

1 pound Brussels sprouts, trimmed and halved lengthwise

6 cloves garlic, minced

salt and ground black pepper to taste

1 tablespoon balsamic vinegar

Directions

Preheat the oven to 400 degrees F (200 degrees C).

Heat oil in a cast iron skillet until shimmering. Carefully place Brussels sprouts, cut-sides down, into hot oil. Sprinkle in garlic, salt, and pepper. Cook until Brussels sprouts begin to brown, 3 to 5 minutes.

Transfer the skillet to the preheated oven; cook until Brussels sprouts are very browned and tender, 10 to 20 minutes. Shake the skillet every 5 minutes to ensure even cooking.

Season with salt and pepper, stir in balsamic vinegar, and serve immediately.

Breakfast Recipes

Greek Yogurt Breakfast Parfait

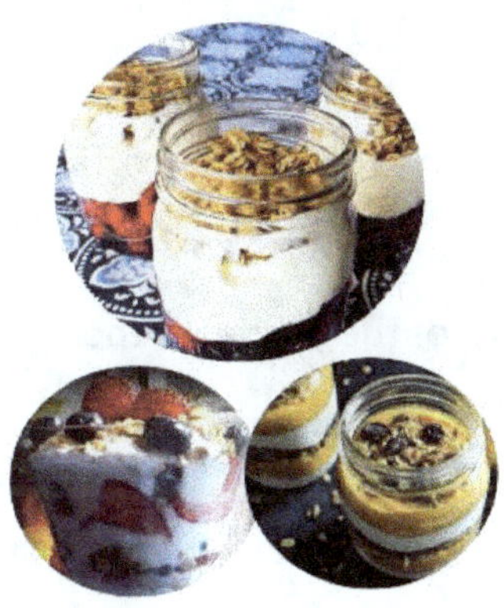

Ingredients

½ cup fresh blueberries

½ cup sliced fresh strawberries

1 teaspoon white sugar (Optional)

6 tablespoons granola, or as needed

1 (6 ounce) container nonfat vanilla Greek yogurt

1 teaspoon lemon zest

Directions

Add blueberries and strawberries to a small bowl. Sprinkle with sugar; stir to coat the berries.

Place 2 tablespoons granola in the bottom of 2 parfait glasses. Spoon 2 tablespoons yogurt on top and sprinkle with 1/2 teaspoon lemon zest. Top with 1/3 of the berries. Repeat layers until the parfait glasses are full.

Spinach Feta Egg Wrap

Ingredients

1 large whole-wheat tortilla

1 ½ teaspoons coconut oil

1 cup chopped baby spinach leaves

1 oil-packed sun-dried tomato, chopped

2 eggs, beaten

⅓ cup feta cheese

1 tomato, diced

Directions

Warm tortilla in a large skillet over medium heat.

Melt coconut oil in a separate skillet over medium-high heat. Sauté spinach and tomato in hot oil until spinach wilts, about 1 minute. Add eggs and scramble until almost set, about 2 minutes. Sprinkle feta cheese over eggs and continue cooking until cheese melts, about 1 minute more.

Transfer scrambled egg mixture to warm tortilla in the large skillet; top with diced tomato. Roll tortilla and leave in skillet long enough for wrap to hold its shape, about 30 seconds.

Spiced Pumpkin Molasses Muffins

Ingredients

1 cup all-purpose flour

½ cup whole wheat flour

¼ cup flax seed meal

¼ cup rolled oats, plus extra for garnish

½ teaspoon baking powder

½ teaspoon baking soda

½ teaspoon salt

2 teaspoons ground cinnamon

1 teaspoon ground ginger

½ teaspoon ground cloves

¼ teaspoon ground nutmeg

½ cup dark brown sugar

1 cup pumpkin puree

½ cup nonfat plain yogurt

2 eggs

3 tablespoons molasses

3 tablespoons unsweetened applesauce

1 tablespoon canola oil

1 teaspoon vanilla extract

½ cup golden raisins (Optional)

½ cup chopped walnuts (Optional)

2 tablespoons pumpkin seeds for garnish

Directions

Preheat oven to 400 degrees F (200 degrees C). Spray 12 muffin cups with cooking spray.

In a bowl, mix together the 2 flours, flax seed meal, rolled oats, baking powder, baking soda, salt, cinnamon, ginger, cloves, and nutmeg until the ingredients are thoroughly combined.

In another large bowl, beat together the brown sugar, pumpkin puree, yogurt , eggs, molasses, applesauce, canola oil, vanilla, and until well-blended. Stir in the flour mixture just to combine, and gently mix in the raisins and walnuts.

Divide the mixture into the prepared muffin tins, sprinkle each muffin with a few rolled oats and pumpkin seeds, and bake in the preheated oven until the tops spring back when touched and a toothpick inserted into the center comes out clean, 15 to 20 minutes.

Lemony Cabbage-Avocado Slaw

Ingredients

6 cups finely shredded white and red cabbage

1 ripe avocado, diced

1 small red bell pepper, chopped

¼ cup shelled hemp seeds

3 tablespoons lemon juice

3 tablespoons chopped fresh cilantro

2 tablespoons finely chopped red onion

¼ teaspoon fine sea salt

Directions

Combine cabbage, avocado, red bell pepper, hemp seeds, lemon juice, cilantro, onion, and sea salt in a large bowl; toss together until slaw has a creamy consistency.

Protein Smoothie Bowl

Ingredients

1 cup fresh strawberries, quartered

½ cup milk

⅔ cup granola, divided

¼ cup blueberries

1 scoop protein powder

1 teaspoon vanilla extract

¼ cup chocolate chips

Directions

Combine strawberries, milk, 1/3 cup granola, blueberries, protein powder, and vanilla in a blender; blend until smooth.

Layer 1/2 of the chocolate chips on the bottom of a bowl. Pour smoothie over top, then sprinkle with remaining chocolate chips and remaining granola.

Blueberry Chia Pudding

Ingredients

2 cups almond milk

6 tablespoons chia seeds, or more to taste

⅓ cup fresh blueberries

1 tablespoon maple syrup, or more to taste

½ teaspoon vanilla extract

1 pinch ground cinnamon

Directions

Combine almond milk, chia seeds, blueberries, maple syrup, vanilla extract, and cinnamon in a blender; blend until smooth. Pour into 3 ramekins or glasses.

Chill until set, 8 hours to overnight. Serve chilled.

Avocado Whole Wheat Pasta Salad

Ingredients

1 (12 ounce) box whole wheat rotini pasta

3 tablespoons extra-virgin olive oil

3 tablespoons white vinegar

lemon, juiced

1 tablespoon honey

2 avocados - peeled, pitted, and chopped

1 green bell pepper, sliced

1 large carrot, cut into matchstick-size pieces

6 green onions, sliced

1 stalk celery, sliced

1 clove garlic, minced

2 teaspoons chopped fresh basil

2 teaspoons chopped fresh parsley

2 teaspoons chopped fresh cilantro

1 teaspoon lemon zest

salt and ground black pepper to taste

Directions

Bring a large pot of salted water to a boil. Cook the rotini at a boil until tender yet firm to the bite, about 10 minutes; drain and run under cold water to prevent sticking.

Whisk olive oil, vinegar, lemon juice, and honey together in a bowl until dressing is smooth.

Mix pasta, avocados, green bell pepper, carrot, green onions, celery, garlic, basil, parsley, and cilantro together in a bowl. Drizzle dressing over pasta mixture and toss to coat. Add lemon zest, salt, and pepper to pasta salad. Serve at room temperature.

High-Fiber Pancakes

Ingredients

1 cup milk

2 large eggs

2 tablespoons vegetable oil

1 teaspoon vanilla extract

1 ½ cups all-purpose baking mix

¼ cup bran meal

¼ cup white sugar

2 tablespoons ground flax seeds

1 tablespoon chia seeds

2 teaspoons baking powder

1 tablespoon butter, or as needed

Directions

Whisk together milk, eggs, oil, and vanilla together in a medium bowl.

Whisk together baking mix, bran meal, sugar, ground flax seeds, chia seeds, and baking powder together in a large bowl. Make a well in the center; add 1 tablespoon egg mixture into the well and whisk until well combined. Continue adding and whisking in egg mixture, 1 tablespoon at a time, until batter has thickened and takes 1 to 2 seconds to fall off the whisk.

Heat a griddle over medium-high heat; grease with butter.

Working in batches, drop 1/3 cup batter onto the griddle about 4 inches apart; cook until bubbles form and the edges are dry, 3 to 4 minutes. Flip gently and cook until browned on the other side, 2 to 3 minutes. Repeat with remaining batter, greasing the griddle with more butter if needed.

Oatmeal with Flaxseed and Berries

Ingredients

10 cups water

1 cup steel cut oats

¼ cup flaxseed meal

¼ cup chia seeds

¾ cup goji berries

¾ cup raisins

¾ cup dried cranberries

¼ cup brown sugar

¼ cup pumpkin seeds

2 teaspoons ground cinnamon

Directions

Bring water to a boil in a large pot. Add oats, flaxseed meal, and chia seeds, whisking well after each addition to prevent clumps. Add goji berries, raisins, cranberries, brown sugar, pumpkin seeds, and cinnamon. Reduce heat and simmer, stirring occasionally, until oatmeal reaches desired consistency, 40 to 45 minutes.

Sweet Potato-Black Bean Quesadillas

Ingredients

5 cups 1/2-inch cubed, peeled sweet potatoes

2 tablespoons extra-virgin olive oil

1 teaspoon chili powder

1 teaspoon ground cumin

1 teaspoon dried oregano

1 teaspoon garlic powder

1 teaspoon onion powder

sea salt and freshly cracked black pepper to taste

4 (12 inch) flour tortillas

2 cups shredded old Cheddar cheese

1 (19 ounce) can black beans, rinsed and drained

½ cup salsa

2 cups shredded Monterey Jack cheese

¼ cup sour cream, for topping

¼ cup chopped fresh cilantro for garnish

Directions

Preheat the oven to 400 degrees F (200 degrees C).

Combine cubed sweet potatoes, olive oil, chili powder, cumin, oregano, garlic powder, onion powder, and a generous amount of salt and cracked pepper in a bowl. Spread cubes out in a single layer on a baking sheet.

Bake in the preheated oven for 12 minutes, stir, flip, and return to the oven to bake until tender, 10 to 12 more minutes. Taste and season with additional salt if required.

Lay out one tortilla on a flat surface and place 1/2 cup Cheddar on one half of the tortilla. Top with a few scoops of roasted sweet potatoes and a generous scoop of black beans. Spoon over 2 tablespoons salsa and top with 1/2 cup Monterey Jack cheese. Fold tortilla over the filling and gently press it down.

Heat a large skillet over medium heat.

Place quesadilla onto hot skillet without any oil and cook until golden brown, about 2 minutes. Carefully flip quesadilla and continue cooking for 2 more minutes. Repeat with remaining ingredients until all 4 quesadillas are fried up.

Slice them in half and serve each quesadilla with a couple dollops of sour cream, fresh cilantro, and additional salsa if desired.

Tart Tropical Parfait

Ingredients

1 (5.3 ounce) container low-fat vanilla Greek yogurt

½ cup chopped kiwi

2 tablespoons chopped macadamia nuts

1 teaspoon agave nectar

1 teaspoon chopped fresh mint

Directions

Spoon 1/3 cup yogurt into a 6- to 8-ounce parfait glass or jar. Top yogurt with 1/2 of the kiwi, 1/2 of the macadamia nuts, 1/2 of the agave. Repeat layers with the remaining yogurt, kiwi, nuts, and agave. Top parfait with mint.

Yummy Veggie Omelet

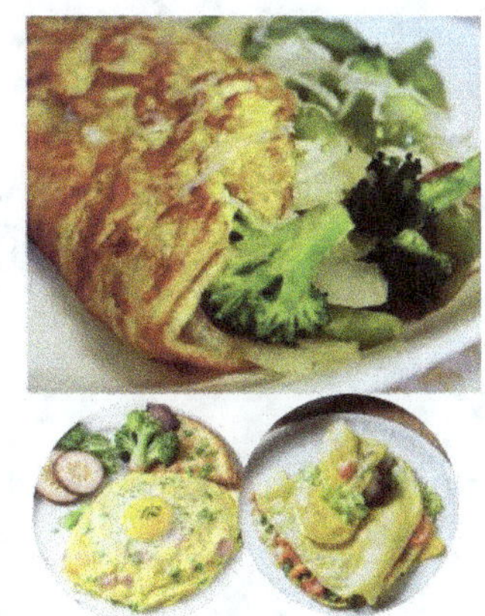

Ingredients

2 tablespoons butter, divided

1 small onion, chopped

1 green bell pepper, chopped

¾ teaspoon salt, divided

4 large eggs

2 tablespoons milk

⅛ teaspoon freshly ground black pepper

2 ounces shredded Swiss cheese

Directions

Melt 1 tablespoon butter in a medium skillet over medium heat. Cook and stir onion and bell pepper in butter until just tender, 4 to 5 minutes. Transfer vegetables to a bowl, season with 1/4 teaspoon salt, and set aside.

Beat together eggs, milk, remaining 1/2 teaspoon salt, and pepper in a separate bowl.

Melt remaining 1 tablespoon butter in the skillet over medium heat; swirl to coat the bottom of the skillet with butter. When butter is bubbly, pour in egg mixture and cook undisturbed until the bottom of eggs begin to set, about 1 minute. Gently lift the edges of omelet with a spatula to let any uncooked egg flow onto the skillet. Continue cooking until the center of omelet starts to look dry, 1 to 2 more minutes.

Sprinkle cheese over omelet, then spoon vegetable mixture over 1/2 of the omelet. Use a spatula to gently fold omelet over vegetables. Cook until cheese melts to desired consistency, about 1 minute. Slide omelet onto a plate. Cut in half and serve.

Lunch Recipes

Pumpkin Hummus

Ingredients

1 tablespoon olive oil, plus more for garnish

2 cloves garlic, minced

1 teaspoon cumin

1 (15-oz can) chickpeas, rinsed and drained

3/4 cup canned pumpkin

1/4 cup water

1/4 cup lemon juice

1/2 teaspoon salt

1/8 teaspoon cayenne pepper

1/8 teaspoon ground cinnamon

1/8 teaspoon freshly ground black pepper

1 green onions, sliced for garnish

Directions

Heat olive oil in a skillet over medium heat. Add garlic and cumin; cook and stir until fragrant, about 30 seconds.

Transfer garlic mixture to a food processor or blender. Add chickpeas, pumpkin, water, lemon juice, salt, cayenne, cinnamon, and black pepper. Blend until smooth.

Transfer into a serving bowl. Garnish with additional olive oil and sprinkle with green onions. Serve with pita bread and cut-up veggies.

Black Bean and Corn Salad

Ingredients

½ cup olive oil

⅓ cup fresh lime juice

1 clove garlic, minced

1 teaspoon salt

⅛ teaspoon ground cayenne pepper

2 (15 ounce) cans black beans, rinsed and drained

1 ½ cups frozen corn kernels

1 avocado - peeled, pitted and diced

1 red bell pepper, chopped

2 tomatoes, chopped

6 green onions, thinly sliced

½ cup chopped fresh cilantro

Directions

Place olive oil, lime juice, garlic, salt, and cayenne pepper in a small jar. Close the lid tightly and shake the jar until the dressing is well combined.

Combine in a salad bowl beans, corn, avocado, bell pepper, tomatoes, green onions, and cilantro.

Shake dressing again, pour over salad, and toss to coat.

Low Cholesterol Turkey Tacos

Ingredients

1 pound lean ground turkey

1 onion, diced

½ teaspoon chili powder

¼ teaspoon garlic powder

¼ teaspoon onion powder

1 cup Mexican salsa, drained

1 (4.5 ounce) can diced green chile peppers, drained

1 tablespoon chopped fresh cilantro, or to taste (Optional)

salt and ground black pepper to taste

12 taco shells

2 avocados, sliced, or to taste (Optional)

1 cup shredded Monterey Jack cheese, or to taste (Optional)

1 cup shredded lettuce, or to taste (Optional)

1 cup diced tomatoes (Optional)

Directions

Heat a lightly oiled skillet over medium-high heat. Saute the turkey and onion until browned, about 8 minutes. Drain and discard juice.

Stir chile powder, garlic powder, and onion powder into the turkey mixture until well combined. Mix in salsa, green chile peppers, cilantro, salt, and pepper. Cook and occasionally stir taco filling until flavors meld, 7 to 10 minutes.

Fill taco shells with taco filling. Top with avocado, shredded Monterey Jack cheese, lettuce, and tomatoes.

Mushroom and Spinach Tart with Cracker Crust

Ingredients

- **Crust:**

½ cup whole wheat flour

½ cup all-purpose flour

1 tablespoon ground flax seeds

½ tablespoon poppy seeds (Optional)

1 teaspoon salt

1 tablespoon olive oil

⅓ cup water, or as needed

- **Filling:**

½ bunch fresh spinach

1 tablespoon olive oil

1 cup chopped onion

1 (9 ounce) package mushrooms, sliced

¾ cup sour cream

⅓ cup crumbled feta cheese

1 egg

½ tablespoon dried marjoram

½ teaspoon salt

ground black pepper to taste

Directions

Preheat the oven to 375 degrees F (190 degrees C).

Combine whole wheat flour, all-purpose flour, flax seeds, poppy seeds, and salt in a medium bowl. Rub in olive oil. Add enough water to make a pliable dough.

Roll out dough on a floured surface and press into an 11-inch tart pan. Poke holes all over with a fork.

Bake in the preheated oven until the surface of the crust looks dry, about 15 minutes.

Meanwhile, bring a small pot of water to a boil. Add spinach and cook until wilted, 2 to 3 minutes. Drain and cool until easily handled; squeeze out all water and chop.

Heat oil in a large skillet and fry onion for 3 minutes. Add mushrooms and continue sauteeing until tender, about 5 minutes. Transfer to a bowl. Mix in spinach, sour cream, feta cheese, egg, marjoram, salt, and pepper. Spread the filling over the prebaked tart crust.

Reduce the oven temperature to 350 degrees F (175 degrees C).

Bake tart until the center is set, about 50 minutes.

Vegan Kale and Chickpea Soup

Ingredients

cooking spray

1 teaspoon minced garlic

¼ cup minced onion

1 quart vegetable broth, divided

4 cups chopped kale leaves

1 (15 ounce) can chickpeas (garbanzo beans), drained and rinsed

1 cube vegetable bouillon

¼ teaspoon curry powder

1 cup almond milk

Directions

Spray the inside of a stockpot with cooking spray; place over medium heat. Cook and stir garlic in the stockpot until lightly browned, 2 to 3 minutes. Add onion and about 2 tablespoons vegetable broth to garlic; cook and stir until onion is translucent, 5 to 10 minutes.

Stir kale into onion mixture; cook until slightly wilted, 3 to 4 minutes. Add chickpeas, remaining vegetable broth, vegetable bouillon, and curry powder; bring to a boil. Reduce heat and simmer until heated through, about 15 minutes. Add almond milk and cook until heated through, 2 to 3 minutes.

Grilled Masala Chicken with Vegetables

Ingredients

¼ cup olive oil

6 teaspoons garam masala, divided

4 small cloves garlic, minced

1 teaspoon salt

½ teaspoon ground black pepper

Reynolds Wrap Heavy Duty Aluminum Foil

4 (5 ounce) skinless, boneless chicken breast halves

4 small yellow summer squash or zucchini, sliced into 1/4-inch rounds

1 medium sweet onion, thinly sliced

½ cup plain yogurt

1 teaspoon Cilantro leaves

Directions

Mix the olive oil, 4 teaspoons garam masala, garlic, salt, and black pepper in a small bowl until combined. Tear four sheets (12x18 inches each) of Reynolds Wrap® Heavy Duty Aluminum Foil. Center one chicken breast half on a sheet of foil; sprinkle 1/2 teaspoon garam masala on both sides.

Place the squash and onion slices on top of the chicken. Drizzle evenly with one-fourth of the olive oil mixture. Bring up foil sides. Double-fold top and ends to seal packet, leaving room for heat circulation inside. Repeat to make four packets.

Grill over medium-high heat in covered grill 20 to 25 minutes or until chicken is cooked through and an instant-read thermometer inserted into chicken registers 165 degrees F.

Open packets carefully by cutting along top fold with a sharp knife, allowing steam to escape; then open top of foil packet. To serve, top with yogurt and sprinkle with cilantro, if desired.

Turkish Red Lentil Soup with Mint

Ingredients

2 tablespoons olive oil

½ onion, diced

1 clove garlic, minced

¼ cup diced tomatoes, drained

5 cups chicken stock

½ cup red lentils

¼ cup fine bulgur

¼ cup rice

2 tablespoons tomato paste

1 tablespoon dried mint

1 teaspoon paprika

½ teaspoon cayenne pepper (Optional)

salt and ground black pepper to taste

Directions

Heat oil in a large pot over high heat. Add onion and sauté until beginning to soften, about 2 minutes. Stir in garlic and cook for 2 minutes. Add diced tomatoes and cook for 10 minutes.

Stir in chicken stock, lentils, bulgur, rice, tomato paste, mint, paprika, cayenne pepper, salt, and black pepper; bring to a boil. Reduce the heat to medium-low and simmer until lentils and rice are tender, about 30 minutes.

Purée soup with an immersion blender until smooth.

Homemade Black Bean Veggie Burgers

Ingredients

cooking spray

1 (16 ounce) can black beans, drained and rinsed

½ green bell pepper, cut into 2 inch pieces

½ onion, cut into wedges

3 cloves garlic, peeled

1 egg

1 tablespoon chili powder

1 tablespoon cumin

1 teaspoon Thai chili sauce or hot sauce

½ cup bread crumbs

Directions

Preheat an outdoor grill for high heat. Lightly oil a sheet of aluminum foil with cooking spray.

Mash black beans in a medium bowl with a fork until thick and pasty.

Finely chop bell pepper, onion, and garlic in a food processor. Stir chopped vegetables into mashed beans.

Stir together egg, chili powder, cumin, and chili sauce in a small bowl. Add to the mashed beans and stir to combine. Mix in bread crumbs until the mixture is sticky and holds together.

Divide the mixture into four patties and place on the prepared foil.

Grill on the preheated grill for about 8 minutes on each side.

Serve hot and enjoy!

Ingredients

1 cup white quinoa

1 ¾ cups water

Dressing:

½ cup Greek yogurt

¼ cup tahini

1 tablespoon lemon juice

½ teaspoon grated garlic

3 tablespoons water, or as needed

½ teaspoon kosher salt

Salad:

1 ½ (8 ounce) packages lacinato kale

2 carrots

2 (15 ounce) cans chickpeas, drained and rinsed

½ cup dried cherries

1 tablespoon olive oil

4 (4 ounce) skin-on salmon fillets

Directions

Stir together quinoa and water in a medium saucepan over medium-high heat; bring to a boil. Reduce heat to medium-low, cover, and cook until tender, about 12 minutes. Remove from heat and keep covered; let sit for 3 to 5 minutes. Set aside.

Stir together yogurt, tahini, lemon juice, and garlic in a large bowl for the salad. Add water, 1 tablespoon at a time, until desired consistency is reached. Season with salt. Set aside.

Pull stems off the kale. Tear the leaves and place in the bowl with the dressing. Shave carrots into long ribbons and add to the bowl. Massage dressing into the salad until fully coated, about 1 minute. Add chickpeas and cherries to kale; toss to coat.

Heat oil in a large nonstick skillet over medium heat. Cook salmon, skin-side-down, until crisp, about 4 minutes. Flip and cook until desired degree of doneness is reached, 3 to 4 minutes more for medium rare. Remove to a plate.

Divide quinoa between 4 bowls. Add the kale salad and top with salmon. Top with a drizzle of olive oil, crack in some black pepper, and serve immediately.

Quinoa Salad with Vegetables

Ingredients

2 cups vegetable broth

1 cup quinoa

3 small carrots, finely diced

2 tablespoons olive oil

2 small zucchini, diced

salt to taste

3 scallions, sliced

Dressing:

4 tablespoons lemon juice

2 tablespoons olive oil

salt and freshly ground black pepper to taste

½ cucumber, diced

7 sprigs fresh dill, finely chopped

Directions

Bring vegetable broth and quinoa to a boil in a saucepan over medium heat. Reduce heat, cover, and simmer until quinoa is tender and the water has been absorbed, 15 to 20 minutes. After 10 minutes of cook time, add carrots and cook for the last 5 to 10 minutes with the quinoa. Remove from heat, drain, and place in a bowl.

While quinoa is cooking, heat 2 tablespoons olive oil in a skillet. Add zucchini and cook, stirring frequently, until softened and browned, about 5 minutes. Lightly salt. Remove and add to quinoa. Mix in scallions.

Mix lemon juice, 2 tablespoons olive oil, salt, and pepper in a small bowl for the dressing; pour over the salad. Add cucumber and dill and toss to combine.

Dinner Recipes

Scrambled Tofu

Ingredients

1 tablespoon olive oil

1 bunch green onions, chopped

1 (14.5 ounce) can peeled and diced tomatoes with juice

1 (12 ounce) package firm silken tofu, drained and mashed

ground turmeric to taste

salt and pepper to taste

½ cup shredded Cheddar cheese (Optional)

Directions

Heat olive oil in a medium skillet over medium heat, and saute green onions until tender. Stir in tomatoes with juice and mashed tofu. Season with salt, pepper, and turmeric. Reduce heat, and simmer until heated through. Sprinkle with Cheddar cheese to serve.

Zucchini Noodle Shrimp Scampi

Ingredients

1 ½ pounds zucchini

¼ cup unsalted butter

2 tablespoons olive oil

1 shallot, minced

2 cloves garlic, minced

½ cup white wine

½ lemon, juiced

1 pound large shrimp, peeled and deveined

salt and ground black pepper to taste

2 tablespoons chopped fresh parsley, or to taste

2 tablespoons grated Parmesan cheese, or to taste (Optional)

Directions

Make zucchini noodles using a spiralizer or julienne peeler.

Melt butter in a large skillet over medium-high heat. Pour in olive oil. Add shallot; cook and stir until tender, 4 to 5 minutes. Add minced garlic; cook until golden, about 2 minutes. Stir in wine and lemon juice; cook until sauce is reduced by almost half, about 3 minutes. Add shrimp, salt, and black pepper. Cook until shrimp turn pink, 2 to 3 minutes. Transfer shrimp to serving plate.

Stir zucchini noodles into skillet. Season with salt and black pepper. Cook until noodles are tender, 4 to 6 minutes.

Return shrimp to the skillet. Stir in parsley and Parmesan cheese before serving.

Vegetarian Shepherd's Pie

Ingredients

2 cups vegetable broth, divided

1 teaspoon yeast extract spread, e.g. Marmite/Vegemite

½ cup dry lentils

¼ cup pearl barley

1 large carrot, diced

½ onion, finely chopped

½ cup walnuts, coarsely chopped

3 potatoes, chopped

1 teaspoon all-purpose flour

½ teaspoon water

salt and pepper to taste

Directions

Preheat oven to 350 degrees F (175 degrees C).

In a large saucepan over medium-low heat, combine 1 1/4 cups broth, yeast extract, lentils and barley. Simmer for 30 minutes.

Meanwhile, in a medium saucepan combine remaining 3/4 cup broth, carrot, onion and walnuts; cook until tender, about 15 minutes.

Meanwhile, bring a large pot of salted water to a boil. Add potatoes and cook until tender but still firm, about 15 minutes. Drain and mash.

Combine flour and water and stir into carrot mixture; simmer until thickened. Combine carrot mixture with lentil mixture and season with salt and pepper. Pour mixture into a 2 quart casserole dish. Spoon mashed potatoes over lentil mixture.

Bake in preheated oven until lightly browned on top, about 30 minutes.

Ingredients

¼ cup sesame oil

¼ cup lemon juice

¼ cup soy sauce

2 tablespoons brown sugar, or more to taste

1 tablespoon sesame seeds

1 teaspoon ground mustard

1 teaspoon ground ginger

¼ teaspoon garlic powder

4 (6 ounce) salmon steaks

Directions

Mix sesame oil, lemon juice, soy sauce, brown sugar, sesame seeds, ground mustard, ginger, and garlic powder in a small saucepan over low heat. Bring to a simmer, stirring until sugar has dissolved. Set aside 1/2 cup of marinade for basting.

Pour remaining marinade into a resealable plastic bag. Add salmon steaks, coat with marinade, squeeze out excess air, and seal the bag. Marinate in the refrigerator for 1 to 2 hours.

Set an oven rack about 6 inches from the heat source and preheat the oven's broiler.

Broil salmon steaks under the preheated broiler for 5 minutes, brushing salmon with reserved marinade. Turn and continue to broil until salmon is opaque and flakes easily, about 5 more minutes. Brush with marinade.

Black Bean Turkey Burgers

Ingredients

1 cup black beans, rinsed and slightly crushed

1 pound ground turkey

¾ cup grated Parmesan cheese

½ cup Japanese-style bread crumbs (panko)

1 egg

1 (1 ounce) package dry onion soup mix

Directions

Preheat an outdoor grill for medium-high heat and lightly oil the grate.

Mix black beans, ground turkey, Parmesan cheese, bread crumbs, egg, and onion soup mix with your hands in a large bowl. Divide into 6 portions and shape into patties.

Cook on preheated grill until no longer pink in the middle, 5 to 6 minutes per side. An instant-read thermometer inserted into the center should read at least 165 degrees F (74 degrees C).

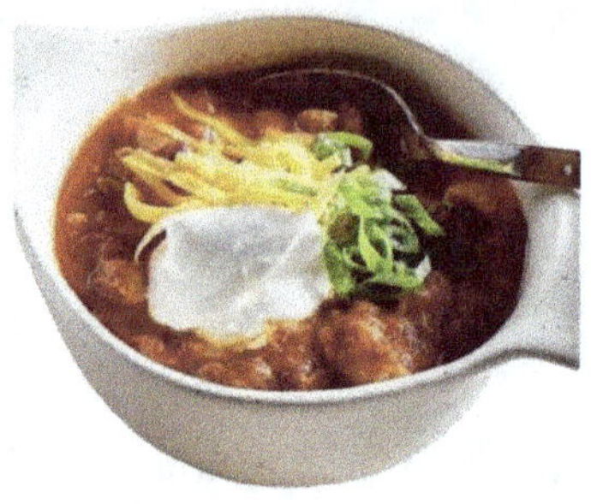

Ingredients

1 ½ teaspoons olive oil

1 pound ground turkey

1 onion, chopped

2 cups water

1 (28 ounce) can canned crushed tomatoes

1 (16 ounce) can canned kidney beans - drained, rinsed, and mashed

1 tablespoon garlic, minced

2 tablespoons chili powder

½ teaspoon paprika

½ teaspoon dried oregano

½ teaspoon ground cayenne pepper

½ teaspoon ground cumin

½ teaspoon salt

½ teaspoon ground black pepper

Directions

Heat oil in a large pot over medium heat. Add turkey; cook and stir until evenly browned, 6 to 8 minutes. Stir in onion and cook until tender.

Add water; mix in tomatoes, kidney beans, and garlic. Stir in chili powder, paprika, oregano, cayenne pepper, cumin, salt, and pepper.

Bring to a boil. Reduce heat to low, cover, and simmer for 30 minutes.

Kickin' Chicken Stir Fry

Ingredients

4 cups water

¼ teaspoon salt

2 tablespoons butter

3 dried red chiles, broken into several pieces

2 cups uncooked white rice

1 tablespoon sesame oil

2 garlic cloves, minced

2 tablespoons soy sauce, divided

1 skinless, boneless chicken breast half, diced

1 teaspoon dried basil

1 teaspoon ground white pepper

½ teaspoon dry ground mustard

1 pinch ground tumeric

1 tablespoon butter

1 ½ cups broccoli florets

1 cup diced green bell pepper

1 cup diced red bell pepper

½ cup diced onion

1 teaspoon lemon juice

Directions

Combine water, salt, 2 tablespoons butter, and red chili peppers in a pot over medium-high heat. Bring to a boil.

Stir in rice, cover, and lower heat to medium. Cook until rice is tender, 15 to 20 minutes, stirring occasionally.

Heat sesame oil in a skillet or wok over medium heat. Cook and stir garlic until fragrant, about 1 minute; pour in half the soy sauce.

Cook and stir chicken, basil, white pepper, dry mustard, and turmeric with garlic until chicken is browned, no longer pink in the center, and juices run clear, 5 to 8 minutes.

Mix remaining soy sauce into chicken mixture.

Cook and stir 1 tablespoon butter with broccoli, green pepper, red pepper, and onion in a separate skillet until tender, about 10 minutes. Stir lemon juice into vegetables.

Toss vegetables with chicken.

Conclusion

In the ever-changing world of dietary habits, the insights gained from studying a low-fat, high-fiber diet are profoundly significant. This diet, which emphasizes reducing fat intake and increasing fiber-rich foods, offers a holistic approach to health that goes beyond simple weight management. As we explore this nutritional philosophy, it becomes clear that the low-fat, high-fiber diet is not just a passing trend but a sustainable lifestyle choice with the potential to revolutionize personal health.

Delving into this diet reveals a sophisticated understanding of fats, distinguishing the harmful effects of saturated and trans fats from the beneficial ones of unsaturated fats. By encouraging the reduction of unhealthy fats and the inclusion of healthier options like nuts, seeds, and avocados, this diet aligns with modern nutritional guidelines aimed at optimizing health without extreme measures or deprivation.

Elevating fiber to a central role marks a significant shift in nutritional priorities. Often overlooked in contemporary diets, fiber becomes crucial for digestive health, weight management, and heart health. This emphasizes the importance of including fiber-rich foods in our daily meals.

The low-fat, high-fiber diet's flexibility and adaptability are key to its widespread appeal. Unlike restrictive diets that may alienate people with different dietary preferences, this approach accommodates various eating patterns. Whether someone prefers a plant-based diet or includes lean animal proteins, the low-fat, high-fiber principles can be easily integrated, making it an inclusive option for diverse tastes and cultural backgrounds.

One major success of this diet is its potential to combat global obesity and related health risks. In an age where sedentary lifestyles and processed foods have led to rising obesity rates, focusing on nutrient-dense, low-calorie foods offers hope. This approach promotes fullness with fewer calories and encourages the consumption of whole, minimally processed foods, aligning with efforts to fight the obesity epidemic.

Beyond weight management, the low-fat, high-fiber diet is a strong ally for heart health. With cardiovascular diseases being a leading cause of death worldwide, our dietary choices significantly impact our heart health. By reducing saturated and trans fats and boosting the cholesterol-lowering effects of soluble fiber, this diet becomes a powerful tool in preventing heart-related issues.

Additionally, the low-fat, high-fiber diet shows promise in reducing the risk of type 2 diabetes by improving insulin sensitivity. The focus on whole, nutrient-dense foods and the benefits of fiber in regulating blood sugar levels align with preventive strategies against insulin resistance, a precursor to diabetes. With diabetes prevalence on the rise, practical and sustainable dietary interventions are crucial.

The adaptability of the low-fat, high-fiber diet benefits various age groups and life stages. From children to older adults, this diet can be tailored to meet different nutritional needs. For the younger generation, it provides a foundation for lifelong healthy eating habits, while for older adults, it helps manage weight, supports heart health, and promotes overall vitality.

In conclusion, the exploration of the low-fat, high-fiber diet reveals not just guidelines but a blueprint for a lifestyle that prioritizes health without sacrificing the enjoyment of food. It highlights that nutrition is not a one-size-fits-all solution but a dynamic journey that adapts to individual needs, preferences, and cultural contexts.

Ultimately, the low-fat, high-fiber diet demonstrates that wholesome eating can be a joyful and sustainable practice. It encourages us to reevaluate our relationship with food, understand the significant impact of our dietary choices on our health, and embrace a nutritional philosophy that nurtures the body, supports longevity, and enhances life quality. As we integrate the lessons from this diet into our kitchens and dining tables, we embark on a path that goes beyond dieting—it becomes a celebration of life, health, and the power of mindful, nourishing choices.

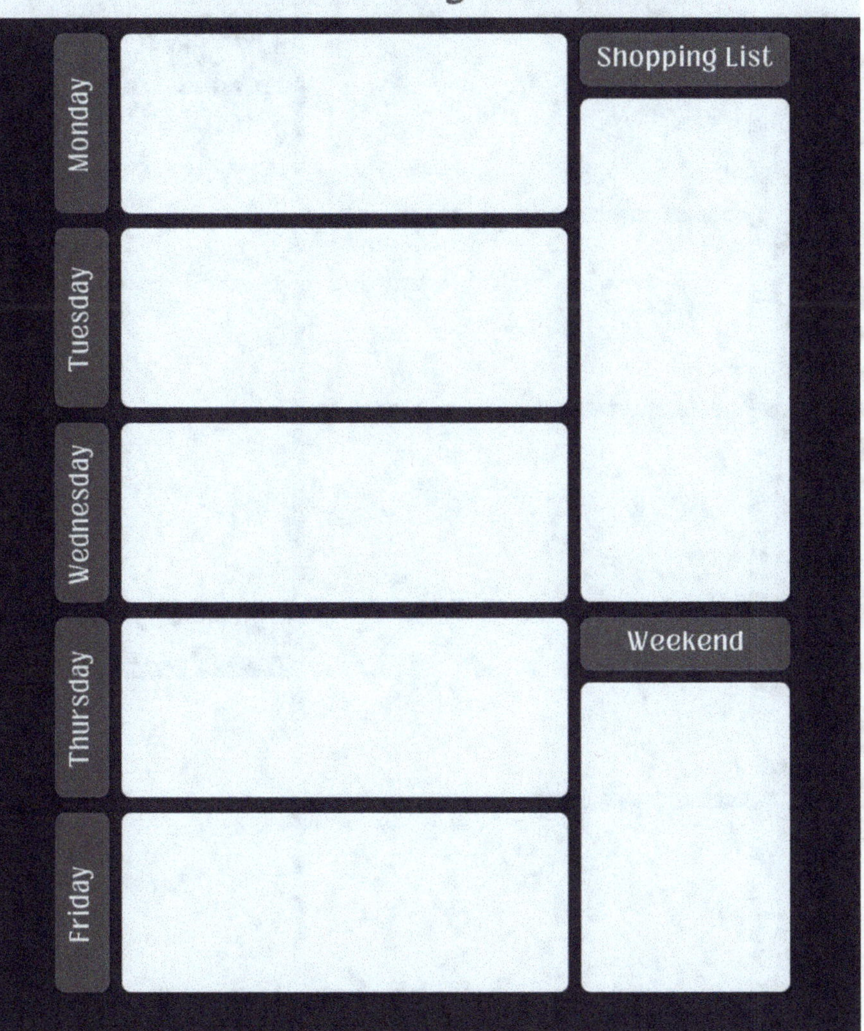
Meal Weekly Planner
Monday
Tuesday
Wednesday
Thursday
Friday
Shopping List
Weekend

Meal Weekly Planner

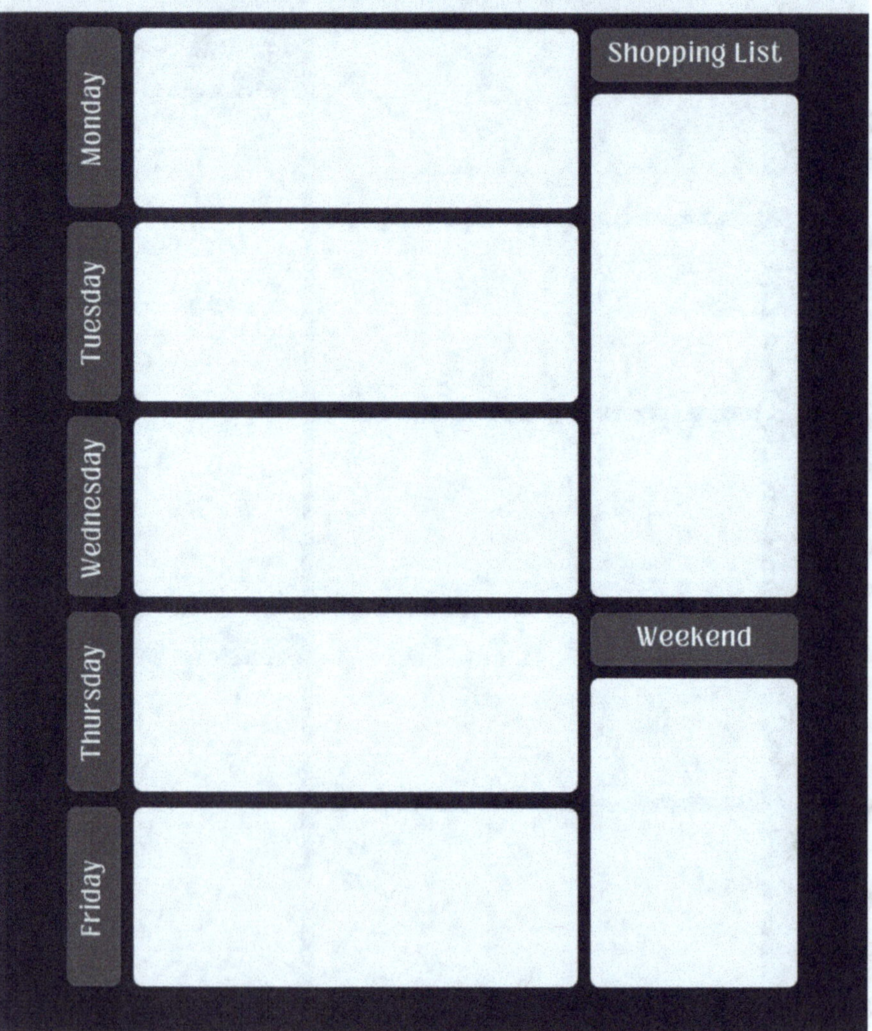

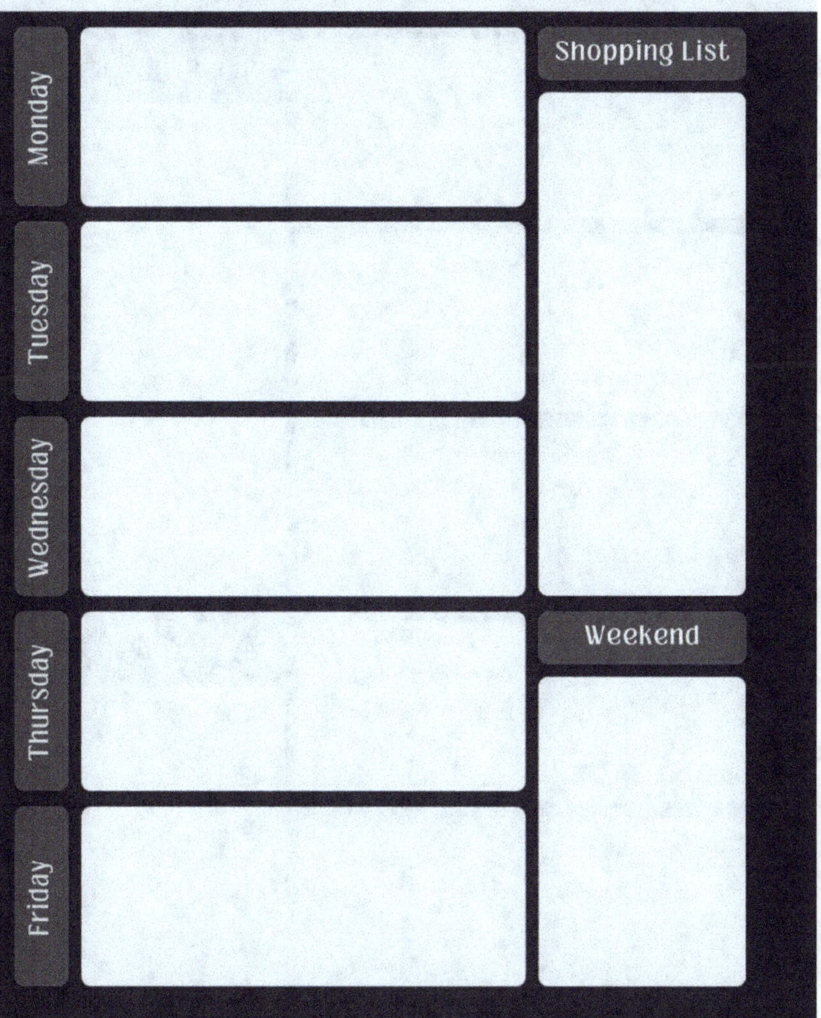

Meal Weekly Planner
Monday
Tuesday
Wednesday
Thursday
Friday
Shopping List
Weekend

Meal Weekly Planner

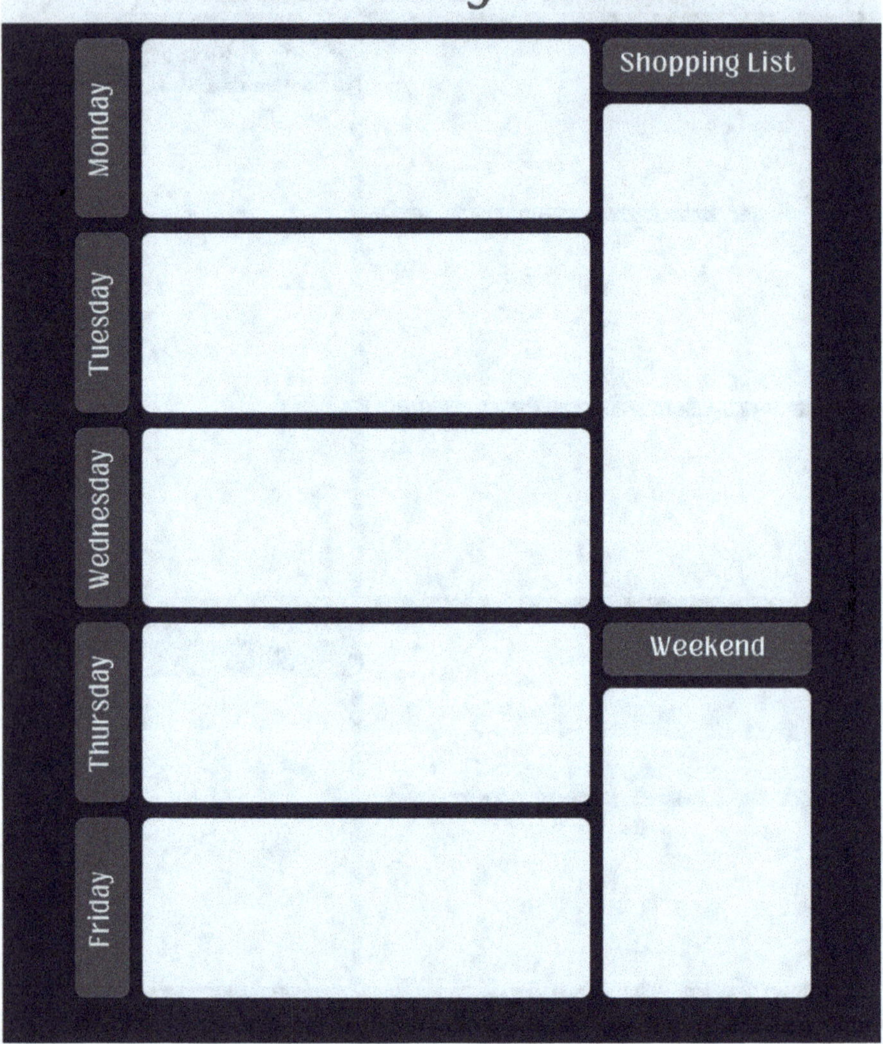